A Journey To An Organized You

This guidebook belongs to:

A Journey To An Organized You

Check Out Our Other Guidebooks

A Journey To An Organized You

Your Step-by-Step Guidebook to An Organized Home

Primary Bedroom

Kandy M. Sartori

Cover and Interior Design by Kandy M. Sartori

OCLLC Publishing books may be ordered through Amazon or by contacting:

OCLLC Publishing
1700 W Market Street, #124
Akron, OH 44313
www.OCLLCPublishing.com

Because of the dynamic nature of the Internet, any web addresses or links contained in this guidebook may have changed since publication and may no longer be valid.

Printed in the United States of America
ISBN: 978-1-960628-00-8 (scbw)

First Edition, February 2023
Second Edition, April 2023
Third Edition, May 2023

Published by OCLLC Publishing

DISCLAIMER: This guidebook contains the opinions and ideas of its author. It is intended to provide helpful tidbits, insights, various viewpoints and informative material on the subjects addressed in this guidebook. However, neither the publisher nor the author is engaged in rendering professional advice or services to the individual reader, and this guidebook is not intended as a substitute for advice from a trained and/or licensed professional. The intent of the author is to offer information of a general nature to help you in your quest for organizing and cleaning your environment. In the event that you use any of the information in this guidebook for yourself, the author and the publisher assume no responsibility for your actions.

DEDICATION

This book is dedicated to you. If you picked it up, there is a reason. Feel free to initially flip through and perhaps you will find your answer or continue into a deeper dive. This guidebook is full of tidbits that have come from decades of organizing, cleaning, self discovery, and detailed observations of what has worked in homes and businesses. The lessons here are from many years of trial and error and simply realizing that every single person knows intuitively what is best for them. It boils down to having the guts to do what YOU want to do. This book aims to be your guide on the on that journey.

CONTENTS

PREFACE

Congratulations on selecting this guidebook out of the many books available on organizing and cleaning. I am thrilled to take you on a tour of your home, uncover thoughts and beliefs that may or may not be serving you, and help plant seeds of encouragement and confidence as you maneuver your way through organizing and cleaning your home.

Listed below is a glimpse of what you will be learning and experiencing in this guidebook:

How to Gain Confidence in Your Purchasing, Decluttering, and Organizing Experiences

- Room by room, you will learn about who you are at your core.
- You will learn how to tap into your inner being and if you have other family members you share your home with, you will learn how to tap into their inner being so you can create the best living environment for every single person in your family, including you.
- Increase your productivity by being organized.
- Learn how to appreciate and embrace your most valuable asset: time.
- Learn how your environment contributes to your health and well being, as well as all members of your family.
- Learn different ways to declutter.
- Learn how to maintain a clutter-free environment.
- Learn how to purchase items that make the most sense for you and your family.
- Learn organizing skills that will serve you in your current home and any future home.
- Learn about outdated organizing ideas that do not serve you or your family.

Organizing comes in many forms. As you walk throughout your day, you may have noticed some things run very smoothly and other areas of your life are filled with hiccups, or hills, or difficulty. Pick your word. Those parts of your day simply are not seamlessly organized as other parts of your day. This organization flows into your home life, your work life, your relationships, and into your body and mind. The most difficult thing in my opinion is organizing our thoughts.

We are raised with beliefs that come from our surroundings and from those that care for us in the best way they know how with the tools they have been given.

As we grow, unless we make some conscious decisions, our friends may remain the same and we may have similar experiences, homes and lifestyles as our friends. The potential friction comes when someone tries to change something in their life and it is different than what their friends and family do or believe. This is quite simple. When we look in a mirror, we see a certain reflection, a familiar reflection. There is comfort in the familiar. However, when we look in the mirror and the reflection changes, sometimes we don't know what to do, how to react, or even move forward. Think of the distorting mirrors in a carnival fun house; some make you laugh, some may scare you, and others are simply interesting. When the people around us see us start to change, sometimes they come with us and sometimes they don't. However, what I can tell you is that as you grow and walk through your own life of mirrors, you will be greeted at every mirror with people who are similar to you. However, going through the process may not always be fun and some of your current relationships may not be the same or even in existence in the future. That is a risk. Is it a risk you are willing to take?

Organizing is a risk. It is a skill that can be learned and needs to be maintained. Learning these skills will involve self-discovery. Self-discovery can lead to change, positive change. As you walk through each area of your home, you will be greeted with the past, present, and future. You will need to work through the emotions that arise. You may need to learn new ways of being in relationships. You may need to learn about boundaries or setting better guardrails. You will learn who you are at your core by working through this guidebook. This process takes years. Yes, you read that correctly, years. I'm not going to sugarcoat the organizing and recovery process. This is a guidebook that you will go through once and hopefully pick up again and go through again in another year or two. Set it on your calendar to do it. You will see and feel changes as you are working through this guidebook but please don't expect things to change overnight. Our thoughts, habits, and beliefs have brought us to this point. We can learn to unpack them and sort out what is truly working for us now.

Of course, this brings up the biggest hurdle of organizing and decluttering: emotions. Emotions play a big role in organizing. In this guidebook we will walk through emotions and various thoughts that you may have or may experience while organizing or donating certain items.

As you read and work your way through this guidebook, please keep in mind the following; "My home reflects every aspect of me. My home reflects who I am today and who I am becoming. I am in balance in every aspect of my life."

What I know for sure is that when our lives are organized on every level, we can live a life with clear, focused thoughts and physical spaces to explore what excites us and create what inspires us.

INTRODUCTION

How do you feel when you walk into a museum, library, or grocery store? When you look around, what do you see?

Now think of your home. When you pull into your driveway, parking space, or simply walk up to your door, what does it say to you? How do you feel? Are you relieved to be home? Does it have the same sense of calm and openness as the museum, library, or grocery store?

We all have a vast background and experiences, we all have gathered some key components/thought processes that uncover our organizing abilities.

If you believe in and look for deep peaceful feelings, then why wouldn't you want your home to have the same peaceful feeling that a museum, library, or grocery store has?

Granted these spaces are designed to hold more people than a home, however I would argue that your home can have the same sense of peaceful calm as well.

Over the years I have been in thousands of homes. When you walk into a home, you can sense the "mood" of the space. Every home has an energy pattern. Every object in your home has energy, whether it is something you purchased, or it was given to you, or left by the previous owner or inherited. Everything has energy.

If you are one of those people who has watched any of the hoarding shows on television and cringed when they toss something out of a second story window and it shatters on the ground, then you are in the right place. You understand energy. Like you, we know objects have energy. A solid piece of wood or even plastic, under a microscope has molecular movement. The object looks firm and solid to the naked eye, but on a molecular level it is still moving.

As you work through organizing your spaces, you will start to feel a flow to each room. It is truly a feeling. As you become more organized and in tune with yourself and surroundings, the more peace and tranquility you will experience. Again, this is a process and it takes time. It is also a never ending process as nothing in our lives is static. Once you achieve the organization you desire, it is simply a matter of maintenance and tweaking. No matter where you move, you will be able to take all the knowledge with you and create organized spaces again and again.

CURRENT FUNCTION AND DESIGN

Let's ponder the current function and design of your primary bedroom. Take this guidebook into your primary bedroom and sit on your bed. Get comfortable and we will take an inventory of the current function and design of your room.

Primary Bedroom Checklist

- ▫ Is this room being used for its primary purpose? Yes / No
- ▫ Do I like the bed? (This is the furniture element.)
- ▫ Is the mattress comfortable?
- ▫ How old is this mattress? (Months / Years) Do I need to think about replacing it? Yes / No
- ▫ Is the floor under the bed clear or is there clutter or storage items?
- ▫ Do you have a mattress pad protecting your mattress? Yes / No
- ▫ Are your sheets comfortable? Yes / No
- ▫ Are your blankets, if you have any, comfortable? Yes / No
- ▫ Do you like your bed cover? Yes / No
- ▫ What kind of comforter do you have? Regular Comforter? Down Comforter? Other?
- ▫ Do your pillows match your bed? Yes / No (King pillows on king bed?)
- ▫ Do you have the right amount of pillows? Yes / No
- ▫ Do you have too many pillows? Yes / No
- ▫ Do you have any window treatments? Drapes / Blinds / Curtains / Other
- ▫ Do you like your window treatments? Yes / No
- ▫ Are your windows clean on the inside, including the window sills? Yes / No
- ▫ Are your windows clean on the outside? Yes / No
- ▫ Do you have a night stand on each side of your bed? Yes / No
- ▫ Lights - Look at all of your light fixtures, do you like them? Yes / No
- ▫ Do you have a dresser? If so, do you like it? Yes / No
- ▫ If you have a dresser, is the top surface pleasing to you? Yes / No
- ▫ Do you have the appropriate amount of furniture in this room? Yes / No
- ▫ Baseboards - Do you like them? Yes / No
- ▫ Light switches and outlets - Do you like them? Yes / No

Primary Bedroom Checklist (continued)

- ☐ Do you like the color of the walls? Yes / No
- ☐ Do the walls need a fresh coat of paint? Yes / No
- ☐ Do you have wallpaper? Yes / No
- ☐ Do you want a different type of wall treatment? Yes / No
- ☐ Do you like your artwork? Yes / No
- ☐
- ☐
- ☐
- ☐
- ☐
- ☐
- ☐
- ☐
- ☐
- ☐
- ☐
- ☐
- ☐
- ☐
- ☐
- ☐
- ☐
- ☐

Current Function & Design

How is this room functioning for you?
How is the layout?
Do you like the design elements?

Current Function & Design

How is this room functioning for you?
How is the layout?
Do you like the design elements?

Current Function & Design

How is this room functioning for you?
How is the layout?
Do you like the design elements?

FUTURE FUNCTION AND DESIGN

This area will be a journal section where you can take notes. If you happen to clear out the entire space, it is a great time to go into the room with a comfortable chair or mat and just sit. Sit in silence or listen to your favorite music and tune into yourself.

- How do you envision this space to be used?

- What enhancements or revisions do you need to make in order for this room to be how you envision it in the future?

We will get specific in this primary bedroom so you can truly visualize your space. Perhaps your space is already the way you want it. Awesome! Move on to the next room. If not, spend some time here. Find magazines and cut out photos of things you like and may want in the room. Do a smorgasbord of all your wishes and wants. Put everything in that appeals to you, even if it doesn't make sense. It may be incorporated in the room you are working on, another room down the road or maybe even tossed aside. If it is tossed aside, there will be a reason why it was tossed aside and that will provide information on your future function and design of other rooms. There will be a flow to your entire home.

Be gentle with yourself and allow your creativity to flow. Write down all of your wishes and desires for the function and design of this room. Don't edit your thoughts, rather, let them flow onto these pages.

Future Function & Design

What are some future enhancements you can make to this room? Are there any design elements you would like to add or delete?

Future Function & Design

What are some future enhancements you can make to this room?
Are there any design elements you would like to add or delete?

Future Function & Design

What are some future enhancements you can make to this room?
Are there any design elements you would like to add or delete?

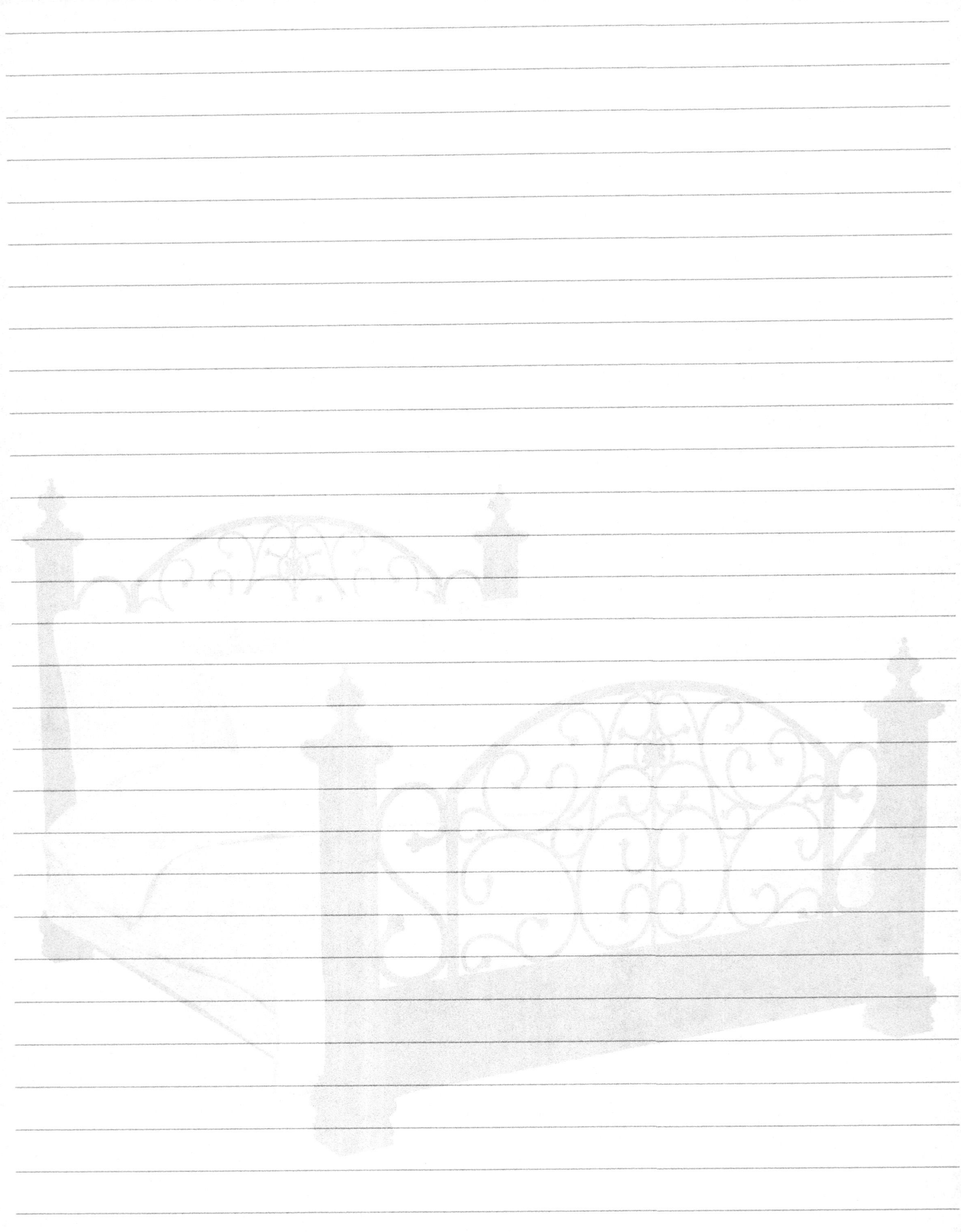

Future Function & Design

What are some future enhancements you can make to this room? Are there any design elements you would like to add or delete?

Future Function & Design

What are some future enhancements you can make to this room? Are there any design elements you would like to add or delete?

Future Function & Design

What are some future enhancements you can make to this room? Are there any design elements you would like to add or delete?

What are some future enhancements you can make to this room?
Are there any design elements you would like to add or delete?

Future Function & Design

Future Function & Design

What are some future enhancements you can make to this room? Are there any design elements you would like to add or delete?

Future Function & Design

What are some future enhancements you can make to this room? Are there any design elements you would like to add or delete?

Future Function & Design

What are some future enhancements you can make to this room? Are there any design elements you would like to add or delete?

CLEANING

This section will be in every guidebook in this series and tailored for each room with the goal for you to form some new habits. We need to see; in this sense I mean, "see" what is in front of us. I have been in many businesses and homes over the years where something may start clean and organized then over time, paper by paper, paper clip by paper clip, and a table here and there appears and before you know it, not only is the room full of clutter, it is also dirty. Of course not everyone is like this. Most people are aware when their home is in need of cleaning, but for some reason, they choose not to clean it. If you picked up this guidebook, the expectation is that either you will clean the space or you will hire someone to clean it for you. If you hire someone to clean it for you, make sure they hit all the sections. You want each room detail cleaned, which means the objects as well. Cleaning the objects and bringing them back to their original beauty will really enhance each room. Not all cleaning companies will do this; most won't but you may find one that will. Otherwise, you may need to clean the object to bring back its vitality.

You may be wondering at this point, "How long is it going to take me to get my home organized and clean?" Excellent question! It all depends upon where you are now and how many people are going to help you, and if you maintain each room once you do get it organized and cleaned. This is the goal. Organizing and cleaning spaces is the easy part in my mind. The harder part is the organizing and cleaning of the mind, body, and spirit. As you go through this guidebook, you may begin to find changes in your mind, body, and spirit. Organizing and cleaning your physical space will organize and clean these areas as well. It's all interconnected.

For example, have you ever walked into a religious building, such as a church, temple, or synagogue? What does the space look like? Is it cluttered? To date, I have not seen any religious building full of clutter, at least not in the main sanctuary. The sanctuaries are generally wide open spaces and there is a peacefulness about them. They are also clean. You get a sense of calmness and tranquility. Which is exactly what our homes should feel like. When you come home each day, you should be excited to enter your home and feel the weight of the world taken off your shoulders. Your home should be your sanctuary. Yes, I used the word "should" quite simply because it should!

If your home is not your own sanctuary, then what is? It's not something out in the future, in a distant land; it is right under your feet. If it is not there now, let's work together and create it. This guidebook will get you there. However, it is not going to happen overnight, over a weekend, or even over a month. Depending upon the thoughts placed into your head as a child and ideas from friends and coworkers, this may be a relatively short or a lengthy process. I know you can do it!

CLEANING (Continued)

There is a part of this process we will talk about in the "Discoveries and Enhancement" phase that took me over six years to formulate. I figured it out after a few years working with my clients but it took me a few more to figure it out for my own family. However, once I did, choices I made about our home are easy to make now. Again, that process took years to figure out.

There have also been things I've learned from a variety of clients who do things very differently than I do. There is not a right or wrong to these differences. That is exactly what they are: differences.

I have noticed however, a very distinct similarity between friends. Your home will mirror your friends. If your home is cluttered, your friend's home is cluttered. If your home is eclectic, your friend's home may be that way too. There may be slight differences but overall you will mirror your friends. This is normal and I hope you choose to create your own home based upon you and your families desires and not your friends or families desires. I can't tell you how many times I have seen a particular gadget or gizmo show up in one house and then friend after friend or family member after family member "has" to have the same exact item. The item can be wonderful for one person but clutter for the rest. Yet, the rest are so afraid to let it go because they will "hurt" their friends or family members' feelings if they don't keep it. Just let it go! If you don't use it or it doesn't fit your style, get it out of your home. Donate it.

As you can see just from this section alone, we may get into the nitty gritty here and there as you go through this guidebook. I will challenge your ideas on things. I will give you the permission you have been seeking to do something. You will gain clarity over your environment and who you are and who you want to be.

It is not going to be easy; I will be up front with you about that but I will be here for you as you progress through this guidebook. You can do it!

Now onto the cleaning section for your primary bedroom.

Cleaning Tools You May Need

- ☐ All purpose cleaner
- ☐ Brass cleaner
- ☐ Floor cleaner
- ☐ Furniture polish (wood)
- ☐ Glass cleaner
- ☐ Granite cleaner
- ☐ Leather cleaner
- ☐ Silver cleaner
- ☐
- ☐
- ☐
- ☐
- ☐
- ☐
- ☐
- ☐
- ☐
- ☐
- ☐
- ☐

- ☐ Duster*
- ☐ Dustpan and brush
- ☐ Microfiber cloths
- ☐ Vacuum with attachments
- ☐
- ☐
- ☐
- ☐
- ☐
- ☐
- ☐
- ☐
- ☐
- ☐
- ☐
- ☐
- ☐
- ☐
- ☐
- ☐

* Dusters: These are for cobwebs. Make sure the pole is long enough to reach all the areas of your room. You may need to purchase a painters pole which will provide the length. Make sure the duster head fits on top of the painters pole.

Cleaning Process

- As you walk into your primary bedroom, either go clockwise or counterclockwise and start from the ceiling and work your way to the floor and out the door.
- Clean the cobwebs (start at the ceiling, work your way around your room and also make sure to go down the wall in the corners.)
- Clean the window pane(s)
- Clean the window sill(s)
- Clean the light switch(s)
- Clean the area around the light sockets, but be very careful. Specifically, the top of the electrical outlets are usually a bit dusty.
- Clean the door handles.
- Check the door above and below the door handles for finger smudges.
- Check the walls for any marks that could be cleaned
- Check out any lights in the ceiling. Clean them safely, if you can.
- Are there any ceiling fans? Again, clean them safely, if you can.
- Clean the baseboards
- Look around and clean any marks on the wall

Cleaning Process (Continued)

- Vacuum the floor including the corners. A vacuum with an attachment is wonderful for this. Yes, even if you have a wooden floor, marble, tile, anything, vacuum the floor.

    - Carpet - vacuum normally using the wand (attachment) in the corners.

    - Non-carpet - You can use an upright vacuum if it has the wand but have it at an angle so the roller brush is not initially on the floor. Go around with the wand and vacuum up all the dust, hair, lint, and any other debris.

- Non-carpet floors - Clean with the proper liquid floor cleaner and wipe up. This may be mopping, microfiber mopping, or hands and knees.

- Next, look at the furniture in the room and start cleaning those items as well.

Depending on what your intention is for the room, you may need to move as many items out of the space and then clean, or if the room is going to stay the same, you can clean as much of it as you can.

Notes on Cleaning

What areas need to be cleaned?
What tools will I need to clean?

Notes on Cleaning

What areas need to be cleaned?
What tools will I need to clean?

Notes on Cleaning

What areas need to be cleaned?
What tools will I need to clean?

TIDBITS

The tidbits section is just that: tidbits or bite sized ideas, suggestions, recommendations, and observations to help you discover how you want your room to function, how to design or modify it, and how to make it fit you and your family.

Think about how you like your clothing in your dresser drawers. Some people like to fold and nicely stack all of their clothing in their drawers. Others prefer to be a little free and don't fold, rather kind of toss their clothing into the drawer. For example, some people will fold their undergarments and others will simply put them in the drawer. Socks are another example, some people have containers for their socks so they stay nice and neat. Others put them all in the drawer. Some color code their socks by using different drawers. Some use different dresser drawers for separating out business, workout, and everyday socks.

How do you like to see your shirts? Most people hang their shirts in their closet, but some people prefer to have their t-shirts in a drawer. Some roll them and some fold them. Most people who are visually oriented tend to hang them in their closet so they can see what they have at a glance. What works for one partner may not be the best option for the other partner. Take each other into consideration when organizing your clothing.

Nightstands. Do you have two? If you are single, consider purchasing another night stand, especially if your intention is to be partnered. Otherwise, you may experience one night stands. Seriously, when you have two nightstands, it does set the intention for a partner and when you do have a partner, they will feel right at home knowing that the nightstand was intended for their use. Yes, this does mean to keep it clear of clutter and not putting anything in the drawers, if there are drawers or shelves. Keep it open for your partner. You may place a lamp, clock, photo, or other items on the top but be mindful of what your partner may like.

Keep the area under your bed free of clutter. The air should be able to flow freely. You should be able to easily run a vacuum or mop under your bed. If you are not able to do this, clear out the items and place them somewhere else in your home. Preferably, you may have a "Staging Area," which is a specific location in your home where you will put items that need a different home or decisions made about them in the future.

Tidbits

As you go about your day, use this section to capture any tidbits you may have that will help you along your journey to having an organized primary bedroom.

Tidbits

As you go about your day, use this section to capture any tidbits you may have that will help you along your journey to having an organized primary bedroom.

As you go about your day, use this section to capture any tidbits you may have that will help you along your journey to having an organized primary bedroom.

Tidbits

Tidbits

As you go about your day, use this section to capture any tidbits you may have that will help you along your journey to having an organized primary bedroom.

INVESTIGATIVE ORGANIZING

Investigative organizing will be ultimately fun and rewarding. However the initial process will tire you if you are like me. I dislike shopping so when I have to go to the store to get all the organizing pieces, then create the jigsaw puzzles and then return the unused parts, it can be a bit exhausting. I'm not going to lie. This process takes time and patience but it is well worth all the agony and the best part about it is that once you do it, you should never have to do it again. If you move, the pieces move with you. You may need to reconfigure a drawer here and there due to different spaces in different places, but overall, once you create your organizing systems, they will follow you everywhere in every phase of your life. If you are in high school and organizing your room, and later your room in college will have the same or a very similar organizing system. When you move into your apartment or first home, you will have the same systems but may need to add a few more. When your family grows, you will need more systems but they will all be similar to the ones you already have. As you move homes and keep "right sizing," your organizing systems will change with you.

This section will be organized so you can count how many organizing bins and containers you need for each drawer, cupboard, and closet in each room. Optimally, you will want to have decorative objects on horizontal surfaces and the rest hidden in drawers, cupboards, and or closets. For example, in your bathroom, it is best to just have hand soap on the counter. Many people will have their toothbrushes, toothpaste, mouthwash, and facial cleansing products on the bathroom counter as well, which simply makes it cluttered and potentially unsanitary if your bathroom counter is one to six feet away from your toilet. The toilet spray can travel one to six feet. Hence, why it is better to store as many items as you can in bathroom cabinets or drawers.

Likewise, other horizontal areas of your home will promote a new you, a reflective you, a family you, and so on simply by the objects you put on them. The idea is to place photos or inspirational quotes or objects on them that bring you peace and tranquility. You want positive and good energy flowing throughout your home.

As I have noted previously, I am not a fan of storage containers and please, PLEASE, do not have winter and summer storage. You don't need it. Combine everything into one closet. When we get to the closet, which is one of the main trouble areas for most people, we will really drill down here so you will not need storage containers for clothing.

Storage bins for holiday items, camping equipment, sports equipment, and a few other groups such as these may work. We will look at these when we get to those rooms, where people generally keep these items in their garage and basement.

One key thing to keep in mind is to make sure that you have enough of certain items in various areas of your home. Every single item in your home will have a space. Sometimes, it is prudent to have more than one to enhance productivity and or efficiency and we will discuss that as well. It needs to make sense for you and your family.

Investigative Organizing

Think about areas that could use a bit more organizing such as a drawer, the top of a dresser or nightstand, or perhaps your jewelry needs organized.
Write your thoughts down here.

Investigative Organizing

Think about areas that could use a bit more organizing such as a drawer, the top of a dresser or nightstand, or perhaps your jewelry needs organized.
Write your thoughts down here.

Investigative Organizing

Think about areas that could use a bit more organizing such as a drawer, the top of a dresser or nightstand, or perhaps your jewelry needs organized.
Write your thoughts down here.

Think about areas that could use a bit more organizing such as a drawer, the top of a dresser or nightstand, or perhaps your jewelry needs organized.
Write your thoughts down here.

Investigative Organizing

Think about areas that could use a bit more organizing such as a drawer, the top of a dresser or nightstand, or perhaps your jewelry needs organized.
Write your thoughts down here.

Investigative Organizing

Think about areas that could use a bit more organizing such as a drawer, the top of a dresser or nightstand, or perhaps your jewelry needs organized.
Write your thoughts down here.

ORGANIZING TOOLS

- **Storage containers for drawers** — All different shapes, sizes, and materials.
    - Determine what kind of material you prefer in your drawers. Some people like clear plastic, some prefer bamboo, some like solid plastic colors, and some prefer wire containers. It doesn't really matter what kind of material you use but it does matter where you put it. For example, a wire container is not the best option in a kitchen or bathroom simply because of the moisture because metal rusts. Meanwhile plastic containers work well for makeup as they are easy to clean up. Determine what works for you in each room. You may have a variety of specific containers for each room, or you may simply use the same style in every room. What matters is that you will use these containers to organize your drawers. These containers can also move with you from home to home as they create systems. Once you create a system, it can flow with you wherever you go. You may have some slight modifications due to drawer sizes, but overall, the systems will still be in place to provide you with a lifetime of organization.

    - Once you identify the container(s) you prefer for a specific room, purchase a lot of them in all shapes and sizes. Purchase way more than you need and keep the receipt as you will be returning the unused ones. Please pay close attention to the store's return policy.
- **Storage bins**, if necessary. To be honest, I haven't been in a single home that doesn't have storage bins, mine included. A goal for all of us is to have none. Holidays are something that some people really get into and each holiday, the decorations go up and then they come down and for some reason, the amount of them keeps growing every year. However, the beauty of working in people's homes is that you find that not everyone celebrates holidays the way you do. Also, some people keep the holiday items on display all year long.
    - Think of the holiday containers you may use for your home. Do you want to color code them? For example, if you celebrate Halloween, would you like the containers to be orange? Containers come in so many colors, you could literally color code all of your containers. If you do decide to do this, I would recommend purchasing all you need at once. Even in a season, the container will change slightly and if you like things neat, orderly, and symmetrical, the slight changes may drive you bonkers and the containers may not stack correctly.

ORGANIZING TOOLS (Continued)

- How many containers do you need? It depends largely on the size of your home. If you have a small home, 500 square feet or less, you may need just one container to hold all of your holiday decorations. If you have a 2,500 square foot home, you will need a few more containers to make it look like you decorated and if you have a 10,000 square foot home or more, you need a lot of containers. How many? Only you can decide that. What looks good to you? I know people who have decorated Christmas trees in almost every room on their main floor. Let's say you have eight Christmas trees on your main floor, you will need a large enough space to store all the trees and decorations. That is quite a few bins and space. Someone who does not celebrate Christmas may have no trees so in essence they will not have a need for as much storage. Hence, they can allocate that space to another use rather than storage.

♦ **Storage for clothing** - No! As I have indicated previously, there is no need for winter and summer storage. Some people who have a home that was built in the 1950's or before may argue they need winter and summer storage bins. I would argue they do not. Hopefully, they have the appropriate furniture with drawers to house a lot of the items one would normally use. Also, if the home actually had a closet, it could be upgraded by taking out the single hanging bar and replacing it with two or three other bars that make the most use of the space. Humans do not need as many clothes as they think they need. Most people do not wear 80% of what is in their closet.

♦ **Hangers** - All the same style. If you prefer plastic, then get all plastic and try to keep them in the same color. If you prefer wooden hangers, is the wood light or dark? What about the hook itself? Is it a chrome finish or something else? Make sure they all match, not only the hanger material and color, but also the hanging hook. This will automatically improve your closet system.

♦ **Label Maker** - You may find adding labels to drawers and shelves may be beneficial.

  - Some parents not only label drawers for their children, they also put photographs of the item on the drawer or container as well. This is especially beneficial as children learn to read.

  - Labeling drawers and shelves is extremely beneficial as you get older and need to hire help. You can label where items go in your pantry, linen closet and even cupboards. As you hire people to assist you, it provides clarity for them regarding where to put the items. The more organized you are, the easier it is for other people to find things.

Organizing Tools

What are some organizing tools, devices and containers you could use? Search the internet for ideas and write them down here along with the store information, price and quantity.

Organizing Tools

What are some organizing tools, devices and containers you could use? Search the internet for ideas and write them down here along with the store information, price and quantity.

Organizing Tools

What are some organizing tools, devices and containers you could use? Search the internet for ideas and write them down here along with the store information, price and quantity.

Organizing Tools

What are some organizing tools, devices and containers you could use? Search the internet for ideas and write them down here along with the store information, price and quantity.

Organizing Tools

What are some organizing tools, devices and containers you could use? Search the internet for ideas and write them down here along with the store information, price and quantity.

Organizing Tools

What are some organizing tools, devices and containers you could use? Search the internet for ideas and write them down here along with the store information, price and quantity.

Organizing Tools

What are some organizing tools, devices and containers you could use? Search the internet for ideas and write them down here along with the store information, price and quantity.

Organizing Tools

What are some organizing tools, devices and containers you could use? Search the internet for ideas and write them down here along with the store information, price and quantity.

PLANNING STAGES AND NEXT STEPS

This area has four quadrants. Each quadrant will correlate to a wall. When your rooms are not square, do the best you can do and what makes sense to you. There are a few additional "odd wall" pages for you to utilize if your room is not square. You will look at each wall and see what you want to keep the same, enhance, or possibly even change. On another page, we will have the next steps and this will also provide a rough timeline. Let's say you have decided you need new sheets, pillows, flooring, and some window treatments.You may be able to do all of this at one time, or you may do it in little chunks one at a time. Perhaps parts of this project are five years out. As long as you envision what you want and put a timeline to it, it will happen. The fun part is planning. As you see things that you like, put them into the Future Function & Design section and relook at your planning stages. If you end up getting a bonus and find something you really like on sale, perhaps you purchase that now.

Keep in mind that as you go through this guidebook, you are more than likely going to start with the room that needs the most attention. Then you will move onto the next room that needs attention. Eventually, you will work through your entire home. As you progress through, your planning stages and next steps could get rather lengthy: and you may need to revise, revise, and revise. You will start to see a clear vision of your future organized home.

Take your time with this section and try to be as realistic as you possibly can so you set yourself up for success. Not only are you going to put it in here, but when the time comes, you will be able to put this on your calendar.

North Wall

Areas To Organize

- [ ]
- [ ]
- [ ]
- [ ]
- [ ]
- [ ]

Areas To Clean

- [ ]
- [ ]
- [ ]
- [ ]
- [ ]
- [ ]

Organizing Tools Needed

- [ ]
- [ ]
- [ ]
- [ ]
- [ ]
- [ ]

Items to Purchase

- [ ]
- [ ]
- [ ]
- [ ]
- [ ]
- [ ]

Items to Relocate

- [ ]
- [ ]
- [ ]
- [ ]
- [ ]
- [ ]

Wish List

- [ ]
- [ ]
- [ ]
- [ ]
- [ ]
- [ ]

East Wall

Areas To Organize

- [ ]
- [ ]
- [ ]
- [ ]
- [ ]
- [ ]

Areas To Clean

- [ ]
- [ ]
- [ ]
- [ ]
- [ ]
- [ ]

Organizing Tools Needed

- [ ]
- [ ]
- [ ]
- [ ]
- [ ]
- [ ]

Items to Purchase

- [ ]
- [ ]
- [ ]
- [ ]
- [ ]
- [ ]

Items to Relocate

- [ ]
- [ ]
- [ ]
- [ ]
- [ ]
- [ ]

Wish List

- [ ]
- [ ]
- [ ]
- [ ]
- [ ]
- [ ]

South Wall

Areas To Organize

- [ ]
- [ ]
- [ ]
- [ ]
- [ ]
- [ ]

Areas To Clean

- [ ]
- [ ]
- [ ]
- [ ]
- [ ]
- [ ]

Organizing Tools Needed

- [ ]
- [ ]
- [ ]
- [ ]
- [ ]
- [ ]

Items to Purchase

- [ ]
- [ ]
- [ ]
- [ ]
- [ ]
- [ ]

Items to Relocate

- [ ]
- [ ]
- [ ]
- [ ]
- [ ]
- [ ]

Wish List

- [ ]
- [ ]
- [ ]
- [ ]
- [ ]
- [ ]

West Wall

Areas To Organize

- ☐
- ☐
- ☐
- ☐
- ☐
- ☐

Areas To Clean

- ☐
- ☐
- ☐
- ☐
- ☐
- ☐

Organizing Tools Needed

- ☐
- ☐
- ☐
- ☐
- ☐
- ☐

Items to Purchase

- ☐
- ☐
- ☐
- ☐
- ☐
- ☐

Items to Relocate

- ☐
- ☐
- ☐
- ☐
- ☐
- ☐

Wish List

- ☐
- ☐
- ☐
- ☐
- ☐
- ☐

Odd Wall

Areas To Organize

- [ ]
- [ ]
- [ ]
- [ ]
- [ ]
- [ ]

Areas To Clean

- [ ]
- [ ]
- [ ]
- [ ]
- [ ]
- [ ]

Organizing Tools Needed

- [ ]
- [ ]
- [ ]
- [ ]
- [ ]
- [ ]

Items to Purchase

- [ ]
- [ ]
- [ ]
- [ ]
- [ ]
- [ ]

Items to Relocate

- [ ]
- [ ]
- [ ]
- [ ]
- [ ]
- [ ]

Wish List

- [ ]
- [ ]
- [ ]
- [ ]
- [ ]
- [ ]

Odd Wall

Areas To Organize

- [ ]
- [ ]
- [ ]
- [ ]
- [ ]
- [ ]

Areas To Clean

- [ ]
- [ ]
- [ ]
- [ ]
- [ ]
- [ ]

Organizing Tools Needed

- [ ]
- [ ]
- [ ]
- [ ]
- [ ]
- [ ]

Items to Purchase

- [ ]
- [ ]
- [ ]
- [ ]
- [ ]
- [ ]

Items to Relocate

- [ ]
- [ ]
- [ ]
- [ ]
- [ ]
- [ ]

Wish List

- [ ]
- [ ]
- [ ]
- [ ]
- [ ]
- [ ]

Item	Amount	Target Date	J	F	M	A	M	J	J	A	S	O	N	D

MONTHLY TO-DO LIST

JANUARY

FEBRUARY

MARCH

APRIL

MAY

JUNE

JULY

AUGUST

SEPTEMBER

OCTOBER

NOVEMBER

DECEMBER

AFFIRMATIONS AND THOUGHTS

This section is for affirmations and thoughts about your primary bedroom. Each room in this guidebook series will have an affirmation and there will be space for you to create your own and to jot down any thoughts. As you work through your room, your affirmation(s) may change little. That is perfect. The affirmations provided will more than likely be the starting point, the trampoline per say, for you to bounce ideas off of and develop your specific affirmation in detail and depth.

One nice thing I learned about affirmations is that after you say it, follow it up with a 100% true statement such as, “My first name is _____.” “My last name is ________.” “I live __________.” “My child’s name is ______.” “My pet’s name is ________.” “The vehicle I drive is ________.” Just make sure it is 100% true. The reason to do this is simple: it is a fact. It is already true. When you are working with affirmations, it takes time for them to really sink in and sometimes they are so far from reality, it doesn’t even seem possible. When you ground them with a fact, they tend to stick. You might find that you may even question the fact. Your fact is 100% true, so how in the world are you even questioning the fact? A good question for you to ponder. This goes to show you the power of our mind. It really likes to play tricks on us so if you find yourself questioning your facts, you may need to modify your affirmation.

If your affirmation feels like you are jumping out of a tall building, then rewrite it. Keep it on your page but tweak it so it feels like you are taking a step off a curb onto the street versus jumping out of a tall building. You may have many affirmations that lead up to your original affirmation. Remember, depending on your goals for your space, this may take some time and effort to reach your goal. Be patient with yourself and enjoy the process.

Sample affirmations could be; "My primary bedroom is peaceful." "My primary bedroom is tranquil." "My primary bedroom is a reflection of who I am."

Use the following pages to capture your thoughts and create your own affirmations that resonate with you.

Affirmations and Thoughts

Use this space to capture your thoughts and create affirmations that resonate with you and your future.

Affirmations and Thoughts

Use this space to capture your thoughts and create affirmations that resonate with you and your future.

Affirmations and Thoughts

Use this space to capture your thoughts and create affirmations that resonate with you and your future.

DISCOVERIES, ENHANCEMENTS, AND NUDGES

This is a space for you to write down your observations and any future enhancements you may want to make to your space after it's organized. It's a great place for you to note what works well, what may need to be enhanced, and most importantly, how you are feeling in the new space.

Everything in our life is interconnected and the more we are in balance with our surroundings, the more we are connected to our inner self. This helps us live our best lives to the fullest.

As time goes on, this is also a section you may return to in a few months or even a few years. Things change in our lives and this area will allow for not only deep reflection on who you were at a certain point in time, but also provide perspective and growth opportunities. Perhaps you feel the nudge to change the theme of the primary bedroom or overhaul the entire space. Pay attention to those nudges. They often start as faint whispers and over time, they keep coming along and pretty soon they turn into nudges. These nudges can be anything from changing the soap in the bathroom to a different brand the next time you need to replace it to moving across the world. While this section of the guidebook is specific to the primary bedroom, you may think that moving to another country cannot even be in the equation, but why is it that when you walk into this particular room you dream of being in a certain country? Do not dismiss what comes up; simply write it down in this section.

If you take the time to revisit this particular section at least once a year and sit with yourself in the room, you will see things coming together. It's like going to the fabric store and purchasing 20 balls of yarn, taking them home, and starting with one strand, knitting it and then taking another and knitting it and eventually, you have created a beautiful scarf. You just didn't quite see it at the beginning.

Enhancements and Nudges

Use this space to capture any discoveries, enhancements, and nudges that you may have about this space.

Enhancements and Nudges

Use this space to capture any discoveries, enhancements, and nudges that you may have about this space.

Enhancements and Nudges

Use this space to capture any discoveries, enhancements, and nudges that you may have about this space.

Enhancements and Nudges

Use this space to capture any discoveries, enhancements, and nudges that you may have about this space.

Enhancements and Nudges

Use this space to capture any discoveries, enhancements, and nudges that you may have about this space.

ACKNOWLEDGEMENTS

Many thanks to the following people for all of their love, support, encouragement, and wisdom.

First and foremost, thank you to my absolutely wonderful husband, Fernando! You always believe in me and you taught me other ways to organize and do things. There is never just one way to do something. You have also taught me that patience is truly a virtue and that balance in all areas of one's life is the key to a good life.

To my wonderful son, Alex. (He may call me his step-mom). Our trip to the local library was life changing. We went looking for a book for school and while we found one for you, I also found a book by an author that ended up being transformational for our family.

To my wonderful coaches, Bernie and Tari. You two know how much your love and support has meant over the years. Thank You is not enough. From the bottom of my heart, Thank You.

To my wonderful WriteSpeak team: Patty N, Catheryn Z, Patrice J, Patty B., and everyone who participated in our discussions. Much gratitude and appreciation to Barbara Sher for her wonderful wisdom and creating a platform for budding authors. This provided so much wisdom and inspiration.

And huge Thank You to Sossi. Your edits and comments were so insightful and encouraging. There is no way this would have happened if it were not for your kindness, patience, and encouragement. Thank You.

I would also like to thank the following people for being a wonderful part of my life and believing in me. Some of the people listed below have no idea how much their communication has meant to me: Albertine, Kay C., Mike S., Lynn & Dave, Rad & Barb, Chuck, Don, Mrs. Nichols, Meri S., Shell B., Mikka B., Emily N., Beth W., Candy C, Candy L, Cindy N, Andy & Danny, MaryKay P., Ruth & William, Margaret & Dean, Tara L., Amy & Tim, Juli and Jason, Anne & Norm, Catherine & Bill, Carol B., Nancy H., Marti N, Bari T., Susie H., Janet S., Pam C., Val S. Dusty W., Megan W. Levi W., Karen A., Guy & Jennifer, Cara & Mike, Doreen & Rich, Pat A., Debbie S., Michael C., Autumn & Willy, Connie K., Brenda and Randy, Sonia and Scott, Hallie H., Megan D., Connie H., Theresa D., Michelle & Joshua, Nancy & Mickey, Heather NW., Michelle L., Judy W., Darrell & Jillian, Charlene R., Marcy T., Amy S., Bruce & Susan, David & Sheryl, Sheryal & Sherrie, and the list goes on. Thank You to everyone who is and has been a part of my life. I look forward to our continued future together.

ABOUT THE AUTHOR

Kandy M. Sartori is a Certified Professional Organizer, serial entrepreneur, author, coach, and Creative Guide. She has over 20+ years working in Fortune 500 companies in positions ranging from Administrative Assistant, Fire/Theft Team Leader, Tax Branch Manager, Financial Advisor, to Bookkeeping. She started her first business in 2009 as an organizing and cleaning business. Over the years, she has developed systems that help her clients stay organized and streamlined.

She works with her clients to tap into their well being. She takes a holistic approach and understands the flow of energy in our lives. She believes that everything and everyone is connected, on every level. She holds a BA in Business Administration and several certificates in a variety of areas, as a true Scanner would. If you don't know who Scanners are or what they do, read, "Refuse to Choose!" by Barbara Sher.

Kandy's motto is, "An Organized Life is a Happy Life™".

Made in the USA
Middletown, DE
06 December 2023

43868098R00086